# The
# Yeast Infection
# Solution

How To Free Yourself from Yeast
Infection… for Good!

Angie S

ISBN: 1499312490
ISBN-13: 978-1499312492

# DEDICATION

For those in search of a reliable and effective yeast
infection solution.

# CONTENTS

# INTRODUCTION

I want to thank you for purchasing this book, "The Yeast Infection Solution".

This book contains vital information about yeast infection and the proper procedures needed to get rid of it. If you are one of the many people that suffer from yeast infection, you may be wondering exactly what it will take to get rid of the embarrassing infection.

Although I know that this is not, in any shape or form, a popular subject to talk about. I realized that there are plenty of people going through the same situation, so my goal is to lead you in the right direction towards finding that solution.

# CHAPTER 1: WHAT IS YEAST INFECTION & ITS COMMON CAUSES?

Yeast infection is an infection caused by the uncontrolled propagation of yeast primarily of the candida genus, a common problem among women. However, in some cases, men also get infected. Another term for the condition is "candidiasis". Normally, a low number of bacteria are present in the vagina. Whenever the population of *Candida* yeast grows abnormally though, an infection emerges.

Candida yeast exists harmlessly in your body particularly the skin and their growth is kept in check by the immune system and other microorganisms in the same area. The most common culprit is the Candida Albicans species of yeast. These yeasts require moisture to grow and therefore prefer areas such as the mouth, armpits, nail beds and genitals, making these the areas where infection is most likely to occur.

Candida infection isn't dangerous except when yeast enters the blood stream and spreads to sensitive organs in the body. Due to this condition being so common; in the course of your lifetime, you are sure to be infected by yeast at least once

Sometimes, an infection only occurs once. However, it is a recurring problem (but with no serious threat involved) most of the time.

## *Causes of Yeast Infection*

Candidiasis can be broadly categorized as either superficial or invasive. The superficial varieties mainly affect the skin and mucous membrane and include oral, esophageal, vaginal, penis, skin and infant yeast infections.

The yeast that causes candidiasis is always present in your body, and is completely harmless unless they it happens to multiply out of control. Certain factors can increase the chances of the yeast growing out of control.

Here are some of the most common causes of yeast infections:

- *Too much moisture*

Wearing the wrong type of underwear, or wearing tight-fitting clothes, doesn't allow the skin to breathe. Fabrics such as spandex, nylon, and other synthetics often lock moisture in the body. Of course, yeasts thrive wherever there's a lot of moisture.

- *Weak immune system*

When a person is sickly, or can't handle stress properly, the immune system weakens. A weak immune system can't prevent the overproduction of yeast in the body.

- *Side effect of medications*

Yeast infection can also be a side effect of taking certain medications, like antibiotics. These medications not only kill bad bacteria, but also the good ones. Good bacteria are needed by the body to stop yeasts from growing in number. They do this by using up the resources required by the yeast to survive.

When we take antibiotics to kill harmful bacteria, the good bacteria that act as our guardians against candida are not spared either. The yeast grows into the areas vacated by the bacteria and begins to multiply.

Other factors that may bring about imbalance of microorganisms include alcohol, steroids and birth control pill usage. Birth control pills and morning-after pills can also cause yeast infections. When a person's hormones are altered, which is what these medications do, the body reacts by letting microbes reproduce freely.

A proper pH balance inhibits the growth of these yeasts and helps to keep their population manageable. A change in body pH levels may thus cause an upsurge in the number of yeasts leading to infection.

- *Poor hygiene*

One of the leading causes of recurring yeast infections is poor hygiene. Make it a habit to regularly change your underwear, sanitary napkin, and tampon – especially when you have a period. Bacteria and moisture multiply throughout the bodies of unhygienic individuals.

It's also advisable to use a tissue, or a wet wipe, after urinating – wiping from the front towards the anus (for the sake of removing bacteria).

- *Irritation*

Using sanitary napkins, tampons, and panty liners that are scented could lead to pH changes throughout the vagina. When a pH imbalance occurs, yeasts begin to thrive. Irritations can also happen when a chemical-based feminine wash is used.

- *Blood sugar is too high*

Women with elevated blood sugar levels, also have higher chances of experiencing yeast infections. The proliferation of yeast occurs when there's too much sugar in the bloodstream. That's why diabetics are prone to recurring yeast infections.

Yeast infections also normally occur before menstruation. The discharge is usually white, odorless, and thick. However, there are also instances in which yeast infections cause discharges similar to cottage cheese.

In rare cases, yeast infection can be acquired from an infected sexual partner. After all, even men can be carriers of *Candida*. Yeast infections, among men, are noticeable because of the reddish appearance of the penis. Though yeast infection is easily treatable, many solutions only work on women.

It is also worth noting that People with seriously compromised immune systems are also highly susceptible to candida infections. People who come to mind include AIDS, cancer, diabetes and psoriasis patients among others. Among AIDS patients, oral and esophageal candidiasis is very common. In fact, AIDS patients account for 50% of people with this type of candida infection.

Angie S

# CHAPTER 2: KNOWING THE SYMPTOMS & DIAGNOSIS

Some common symptoms of candidiasis include changes in mucous membrane, foul smelling liquid discharges and irritation in affected areas. However the symptoms tend to vary according to the type of infection one is suffering.

Oral candidiasis can be identified by the presence of a yellow or cream coating on the tongue and mouth known as thrush. Other symptoms may include discolored patches on the tongue and palate, red or pink blotches on the palate as well as red cracks at the corners of the mouth.

Perhaps the most well known and most common type of yeast infection is that which affects the vagina. Vaginal yeast infections, as suggested by the name affect the female genitalia and are of course specific to women. It is a very common condition. In fact 3 out of 4 women have it in varying degrees of severity in the course of their lifetimes.

## *Yeast Infection in Women*

These are the common symptoms experienced by women:

- Itchiness (in the vaginal region)
- Redness and irritation, particularly on the vulva
- White, odorless, thick discharge
- Burning sensation while urinating or having sex

If you spend a lot of time with your hands in water, you may get candidiasis of the finger nails. It manifests as red, swollen areas around the nails and is accompanied by considerable pain. In more severe cases, it may lead to separation of fingernails, exposing a discolored nail bed.

Infant yeast infection may occur in babies who are delivered or breastfed by infected mothers. You can detect infection on your baby by looking for red patches that look like diaper rashes. if the rash doesn't disappear within a week this should give you sufficient cause for suspicion and you should have your child examined by a doctor.

## *Yeast Infection in Men*

In some cases, men suffer from yeast infection too. However this condition is much rarer compared to its prevalence among women.

These are the common symptoms men experience:

- Penile itching
- Redness (throughout the tip of the penis)
- Burning sensation (especially while peeing)

- Thick discharge under the foreskin
- Change in odor (often a foul, fishy smell)

The presence of these symptoms may indicate yeast infection. However, these also serve as symptoms of other illnesses (such as those that affect both reproductive and urinary systems). When in doubt, it is still best to consult your doctor.

Here are some questions that your doctor will most likely ask:

- Have you taken any medication lately?
- What activities have you done in the past week?
- Are you sexually active?
- Does your sexual partner have an infection?

Your doctor may also run several tests. That means you might be required to have your blood taken (to check your glucose levels). It's also possible that your doctor would perform a swab test that involves taking samples from the inflamed area (to find out whether there's an abundance of microbes).

Penile yeast infections happen because of the following reasons:

- Poor hygiene
- Uncircumcised (microorganisms thrive in the foreskin)
- Acquired from sexual partner
- Skin irritation caused by fragrant body soaps

A yeast infection is relatively easy to treat. It can also stop on its own. Some doctors prescribe pills, creams, and antibiotics to combat the infection.

Yeast infection can be a recurring problem for people who have poor hygiene and high levels of sugar. As also pointed out, yeast infections can be caused by another illness, such as diabetes. So, consult your doctor about your other ailments. By solving those health concerns first, your chances of permanently ending your infection would greatly increase.

If you are obese or pregnant you are at a higher risk of getting a yeast infection. Obese people have more folds in their skin and sweat more creating excellent conditions for yeast to grow. Pregnant people usually experience temporary obesity and their immune systems are weakened, which increases the chances of getting infected.

# CHAPTER 3: DEBUNKING THE MYTHS ASSOCIATED WITH YEAST INFECTION

Below are the popular myths associated with yeast infection:

- *Yeast Infection can only stopped by taking oral medication*

This is not true. Not all oral medications can stop a yeast infection. In fact, the population of yeast grows after taking certain pills. Yeast is also able to adapt to antibiotics.

- *It only occurs to women*

This is false. Women are most likely to experience yeast infections, but men can also be infected. Yeast infections occur among men whenever their penises are irritated or become reddish. The term used to describe *Candida*-induced infections among men is "penile yeast infection".

- *Yeast infection is a Sexually Transmitted Disease*

Yeast infection is not an STD. In fact, it can happen to girls who haven't reached puberty. It can also affect those who haven't experienced sex yet. Similar symptoms may appear on people who have STDs, but the treatments carried out for them are both different and complex. To know for sure whether you really have a yeast infection, simply consult a doctor

- *Anti-Candida Diets can eliminate yeast infections*

Avoiding foods that trigger accelerated yeast reproduction will not cure you. Instead, the anti-*Candida* diet will only temporarily relieve the symptoms and pain. It can lessen the itching and soreness for a while. Though the anti-*Candida* diet helps, it doesn't solve the root cause of the problem.

- *It is caused by heavy metal*

It is a common belief that exposure to heavy metals causes yeast infection. For example, it's a myth that tooth fillings lead to mercury poisoning. Long and increased exposure to mercury can weaken the immune system, but it isn't the direct cause of yeast infection.

- *It is not life threatening*

Complications may arise when a yeast infection's untreated. The microbe may grow rapidly and get into the bloodstream, which in turn harms the body. Also, serious yeast infections (such as those that manifest in the mouth and in the esophagus) can interfere with normal breathing and eating. Obviously, those who have such conditions need to be hospitalized.

- *If it gets itchy down there, it's automatically a yeast infection*

This is false. Many kinds of bacterial vaginosis have symptoms similar to those caused by candidiasis. It's best to consult your doctor, and undergo a swab test to identify the problem.

- *Yeast infections only affect the reproductive organ*

Yeast infections can also spread to the mouth area and the esophagus. As previously mentioned, these type of infection are often more serious and require immediate treatment.

- *Probiotics cure Candida*

Probiotics cannot cure yeast infections. It can only prevent *Candida* from invading the body, if it hasn't yet. When an infection is already present, it is not advisable to take probiotics – doing so might lead to much faster yeast reproduction.

- *Oxygen can eliminate yeast infection*

This is not true. Yeasts are more than capable of thriving in exposed areas, like the mouth. Oxygen cannot kill *Candida.*

- *Yeast infections can be passed on while swimming*

Swimming pools contain chemicals that kill any microbe that's present in the water. These chemicals can also kill *Candida*, which in turn makes it impossible for a person with yeast infection to infect other people in the pool.

However, after taking a swim, immediately change your underwear and clothes. Wet and damp clothing triggers yeast infections. Remember, *Candida* thrives in most moist places.

# CHAPTER 4: HOW TO PROPERLY TREAT YEAST INFECTION

Because the symptoms of yeast infection are so typical, sufferers of yeast infections often self-diagnose and self-medicate. The risk here is that the infection will be incorrectly diagnosed and treated. There are a number of different infections which may mimic a yeast infection and these will require alternative treatments.

In actual fact, the Journal of Obstetrics and Gynecology in 2002, reported a study where only 33% of woman who were self-treating for vaginal thrush actually had a yeast infection. All the rest were infected by other pathogens which needed alternative medication.

When a yeast infection does not disappear and keeps recurring, it might be time to consult your doctor. Doctors often prescribe creams and oral medications.

*Three Commonly Prescribed Treatments for Yeast Infection*

- *Anti-Fungal Vaginal Creams (AFV)*

When there there's an abundance of yeast in the vagina, the doctor will prescribe creams. Stronger medicated creams are taken for shorter periods. Certain creams contain steroids to stop inflammations, and thus are applied only for several days.

Popular brands of AFV creams are Terazol and Micatin.

For men, a cream known as Nystatin works in eliminating penile yeast infection.

These creams often come with tools that aid in measuring the amount to be applied. It is important to strictly follow your doctor's prescription. If ever you run out of topical antimicrobials and yet there is still an infection, you should consult your doctor again. Do not self-medicate since it can worsen your yeast infection.

- *Oral Medications*

Oral medications are given to people who experience recurring yeast infections. Doctors normally prescribe Diflucan and Ketoconazole. These medications are taken under the doctor's supervision. Unfortunately, yeast-fighting pills trigger side effects – such as stomach discomfort, dizziness, and headache.

Taking oral medications is a fast and effective way to kill the yeast in your body.

However, Ketoconzole should not be taken for long periods, because doing so damages the liver. Here's an interesting fact though – both men and women usually benefit from the same kind of oral medications.

- *Vaginal Suppository*

Suppositories are a great alternative if you don't want to take oral medication. It is also safe to use for pregnant women. Popular brands such as "Yeast Away" and "Yeast Arrest" are effective in treating infections.

Usually, a suppository is used before bedtime. Once inserted in the vagina, it will melt. It is also advisable to wear an overnight pad, because suppositories tend to leak. To prevent the leak from staining your bed sheet, place a towel or blanket above your sheets.

There is no penile suppository available. Only creams and oral medications can be used when it comes to treating men. When the penile yeast infection subsides, the doctor may advise uncircumcised men to undergo circumcision. Uncircumcised men are prone to recurring penile yeast infections because microbes proliferate in the foreskin.

In some cases, the doctor will not prescribe any medication or cream. Instead, the patient will simply be advised to practice good hygiene and wait for the infection to heal. If the yeast infection is not that severe, the vagina (or penis) can heal on its own.

## *What are The Restrictions?*

While undergoing a course of medications, several activities are prohibited – these include the following:

- *Abstain from sex*

When under any medication (even creams and suppositories), it's best not to engage in sexual intercourse.

Having creams or suppositories in the affected region will only make sex messy and unsatisfying. In addition, there is the possibility of worsening the condition (due to friction).

If you must really engage in sexual acts, at least, use protection. This may lower the risk of worsening the problem at hand – nothing's guaranteed though.

- *Avoid the ingredient Nonoxynol-9*

This is an ingredient used as a spermicide in condoms and lubricants. This encourages yeasts to grow in number. If the need for lubricants arises, look for a non-perfumed mineral oil product.

- *Cut down on sugar or sweet foods*

Yeast grows rapidly in sugary surroundings. Skip the chocolate bar and cut down your intake of fruits. Sugars from these foods will literally feed the yeasts, further increasing their population

- *Stay away from alcoholic beverages*

Yeast is a common ingredient among alcoholic beverages, especially beer. When the body absorbs alcohol, it is transformed into sugar. As you've learned, this will only make *Candida* thrive even more.

- *Avoid tight clothing*

These clothing ranges from skinny jeans to thongs (anything made from spandex). Allow your skin to breathe. It's advisable to wear cotton underwear and loose clothing.

- *Take a break from using chemical-based feminine wash*

Instead of using a harsh feminine wash, use a natural (or organic) soap to cleanse your vagina. Warm water alone can also be used. The vagina has a natural way of cleaning itself.

- *Avoid scented sanitary napkins, panty liners, or tampons*

Choose a fragrance-free napkin or tampon instead. The chemicals used to add fragrance to napkins worsen yeast infections.

- *Avoid wearing nylon pantyhose or spandex leggings*

These materials retain moisture in the body. Opt for cotton, which keeps moisture away from the body.

Angie S

# CHAPTER 5: NATURAL HOME REMEDIES FOR TREATING YEAST INFECTION

When treating yeast infection for the first time most sufferers use prescription or over-the-counter topical medications. But for many folks the infection just returns at some later stage. Recurring yeast infection can happen because these drug-based medications just attack the local symptoms, not the root cause.

So in turn, many sufferers of recurrent yeast infections have turned away from using pharmaceutical preparations because they are concerned about the effects of their frequent use. A large number of frequent yeast sufferers are now turned to simple but effective natural home remedies

Whether you are experiencing a yeast infection for the first time or it's a recurring problem, these home remedies will help improve your condition. It can eliminate yeast infection in a natural way. Also, these remedies are cheap and easy to make. These are also safe for pregnant women.

## *List of Natural Home Remedies:*

- *Yogurt*

Yogurt is the most popular home remedy to treat and cure yeast infections. Yogurt is a natural source of lactobacillus acidophilus which is a good bacteria that will create an acidic environment the candida bacteria cannot live in. Supplying your body with extra acidophilus should be a part of any treatment for yeast infections.

For yogurt to be used as a treatment it must be plain non-flavored with no sugar or fruit added. You should include a cup of yogurt for breakfast each day until a full week after all your yeast infection symptoms are gone. Women can add a few tablespoons of fresh yogurt to their vaginal area or they can use a tampon basted with yogurt and insert it into the vagina

- *Use scent free or mild soaps*

It's nice to give your body a break from the usual cleansing bar. Those are often filled with chemicals that alter the body's normal PH. Use mild soaps to wash your body several times a day. It'd also be better if you can find ones that are labeled "organic".

- *Dry yourself well*

After taking a bath, wipe your body until it's completely dry. Use an unscented tissue to wipe your vagina. Do keep in mind that yeast thrives in dark, moist areas.

- *Wipe yourself*

After urinating, wipe from the vagina to the buttocks to

remove bacteria. You can use toilet paper or unscented feminine wipes

- *Drink cranberry juice*

Cranberry juice helps lower the pH of urine. Drink one to three glasses of cranberry juice to hasten the removal of yeast.

- *Boric Acid Capsules*

These are a cheap alternative to suppositories. Insert the capsule to the vagina and wait for it to melt. You could also remove the pill's contents and rub it directly on the affected area

- *Use Garlic*

Garlic can be eaten in its raw form, or you can add it to your meals. Well-known anti-bacterial and anti-fungal properties can be found in garlic. After yogurt, garlic is the leading home remedy choice for yeast infections.

You can also rub a small amount of garlic on the affected area. Garlic has properties that kill bacteria instantly. Another option is to use garlic capsules – take them orally, or as a vaginal suppository.

- *Use rosemary or thyme*

Go the natural way by boiling one teaspoon of rosemary (or 1 teaspoon thyme) mixed together with a cup of water. You can drink this concoction, or allow it to cool and use it to wash the infected area.

- *Salt & Vinegar bath*

Fill your bathtub with water, and then add half a cup of vinegar and half a cup of salt. Then stay in the tub for 15 to 20 minutes. The disinfecting properties of salt and vinegar will kill the bacteria. White vinegar and apple cider may be also used for this solution.

- *Vinegar wipes*

Combine two to four teaspoons of vinegar with a pint of water. Use a clean cloth (or a piece of disposable tissue), soak it in the vinegar mixture and wipe the affected area. Men can also use this mixture to wipe the infected part of their penises.

- *Use a hairdryer*

After taking a bath, use a blow dryer to thoroughly dry your crotch area. Put the blow dryer in cool, or low, setting. Afterwards, position it two inches away from the crotch area. This is to ensure no moisture is present where the yeast could thrive

- *Use Tea Tree Oil to create your own douche wash*

You can use tea tree oil or apple cider vinegar. These ingredients contain anti-inflammatory and anti-microbial properties. To make your own wash, dissolve a drop of tea tree oil in a tablespoon of water. As for using vinegar, simply mix a tablespoon of it with a pint of $H_2O$. An alternative way of using these solutions is by wetting a cotton ball, and gently rubbing affected area with it.

- *Epsom Bath*

Fill your tub with warm water, and add half a cup of Epsom salt. Stay in the tub for 15 to 30 minutes to ensure that maximum contact with the Epsom salt. That substance contains magnesium, which kills bacteria and eliminates toxins

- *Lemon water*

Lemon contains acid. It aids in normalizing the pH of the body. Add two to three teaspoons of lemon juice to your tea during breakfast. You could also fill a pitcher with water and add sliced lemon to it – this will alter the water's PH.

- *Buy alkaline water*

Choose alkaline water over distilled or mineral. Alkaline has properties that normalize the acidity of the body. This also eliminates the presence of yeast from the body.

- *Rehydrate*

Drink at least eight glasses of water daily to flush out yeast from the body. Water removes the impurities of in your body by forcing you to urinate.

- *Change towels everyday*

Yeasts may thrive on your bath towel. It's best to change your bath towel on a daily basis. Allow your towels to be sun-dried too.

- *Laundry clothes in hot water*

When your clothes are in the washing machine, choose the "hot cycle" option to kill microbes. If you are hand washing your underwear, you can pour hot water on it (don't move it for at least 15 minutes).

- *Use liquid soap*

Avoid infecting other people by using a liquid body wash. This will ensure the microorganisms won't be transferred to others, particularly those you're sharing toiletries with.

- *Use coconut oil*

Coconut oil has anti-inflammatory properties that will helps stop inflammation. Apply it directly on the affected area. It is not advisable to drink coconut juice because it usually contains lots of sugar. As mentioned, sugar causes yeast to proliferate.

- *Use oregano*

Oregano capsules, or oregano oil, can be used for treatment. The capsules can be taken orally both by men and women. It can also be used as a suppository. Mix oregano oil with both water and olive oil to create a solution, which can be directly applied to inflamed areas.

- *Use aloe vera*

Aloe vera gel has antimicrobial and anti-inflammatory properties. Both men and women can use aloe vera gel to feel relief

- *Use honey*

Though honey is high in sugar, its antimicrobial properties will kill the yeast. Apply directly to the affected area, allow it to sit for ten minutes. Wash thoroughly, and dry completely. Do this several times a day.

- *Use gentian violet*

Gentian violets are available in most local pharmacies. It is used to treat fungal problems. Wet a cotton swab with gentian solution, and then apply lightly on the affected area. Do this twice or thrice a day, for at least a week.

- *Incorporate calendula in your diet*

Calendula is a flower traditionally used for cooking, and known for its medicinal benefits. Interestingly though, it has anti-inflammatory properties and it can eliminate yeast infections. It can be eaten as part of a salad. The petals can be boiled, taken as a beverage.

The benefit of using these natural medications is that they are cheap, readily available and can be used in any combination. This allows for the rotation of medications so that resistance to the natural medication does not develop. Because the medications are natural they are safe to use with very few side effects.

It is important to have a holistic approach to treating yeast infections so the other important consideration when treating recurrent yeast infections is diet. It is estimated that approximately 80% of recurrent yeast infections are affected by diet. It is important therefore to make dietary changes when treating recurrent yeast infections.

Angie S

# CHAPTER 6: THE BENEFITS OF EATING HEALTHY

A healthy lifestyle is the key to preventing yeast infections from recurring. People who follow a balanced diet, exercise regularly, and manage stress efficiently have lesser chances of suffering from yeast infections.

If you have a yeast infection, keep this food percentage rules in mind:

- 60% high-fiber
- 25% high-protein
- 10% complex carbohydrates
- 5% fruits (natural sugars).

The ideal food intake should consist of high-fiber foods, along with high-protein ones. You shouldn't get too much carbohydrates, you have to keep your sugar intake minimal. A healthy person has a strong immune system that could kill bad most microbes. It's important to remember that good bacteria are also present in the body. These good bacteria play an important role in keeping bad bacteria under control.

### *Foods That Should Be Consumed:*

- *High Fiber food*

These foods contain fiber, which is essential in lowering both blood sugar and cholesterol levels. Some example of high-fiber foods include corn, black beans, avocado, chickpeas (garbanzo), brown rice, snow peas, vegetables (garlic, ginger, and broccoli), pear artichoke, oatmeal (rolled or quick), kale and cabbage.

Whole-wheat products like bread, flour, and pasta are good sources of fiber too.

- *High Protein*

These foods aid weight-loss endeavors and promote a healthy diet. Here are some example of high-protein foods – salmon, beef, white meat (chicken or turkey), fish, pork (choose healthy cuts), eggs, low-fat dairy products (cheese and milk), beans, and whole-wheat products.

- *Complex Carbohydrates*

These are some examples of complex carbohydrates foods – whole-grain breads, beans, and starchy vegetables. Starchy vegetables include the squash, parsnips, potato, and sweet potato

- *Natural Sugars*

All fruits contain natural sugars, so eat fruits in moderation. This natural sugar may lead rapid yeast reproduction. Choose vegetables over fruits as a source of vitamins and anti-oxidants.

These simple eating choices could help you stay yeast free for life.

## *Foods to Avoid*

The eats and drinks in the list below are not suitable for people suffering from yeast infections. It's best to completely avoid these (or at the very least, limit consumption).

Of course, sugar is first on the list.

Refined sugar is a breeding ground for yeast. It is almost present in every food such as white bread, white rice, and white pasta. Always remember that it's smart to stay away from "white" foods. By the way, sugar is also found in corn syrup, honey, molasses, date syrup, and maple.

You should also be on the lookout for the following ingredients when buying processed or canned foods – sucrose, fructose, lactose, glycogen, glucose, monosaccharide and polysaccharides. These ingredients are simply other terms for sugar.

Other foods to be avoided:

- *Alcohol*

Alcoholic beverages contain yeast, especially beer. It is a breeding ground for *Candida*. Alcohol also weakens the immune system, making the body vulnerable to infection.

- *Fermented or Processed Drinks*

Stay away from processed drinks because they are high in sugar. This also includes caffeinated beverages (like coffee, root beer, and cola).

- *Processed Food*

These foods contain chemicals that worsen yeast infections. Smoked meat (salmon and sausages), beef jerky, bacon, and hotdog are just a few examples of highly processed foods.

Stay away from canned goods too. It is likely that they contain yeast, refined sugars, and other chemicals that aggravate the infection.

- *Moldy or Aged Cheese*

These cheeses, including processed ones, can worsen yeast infections.

- *Nuts*

Stay away from nuts (pistachio, cashew, etc). Nuts contain molds that are not visible to the naked eye. They also allow *Candida* to rapidly grow in number.

- *Yeast*

Keep away from foods that contains yeas – these may include bread and beer. Consuming almost anything with yeast will worsen your infection.

- *Condiments*

Dips and sauces (such as mayonnaise, mustard, ketchup, BBQ sauce, and processed salad dressing) should all be avoided. These contain sugars and preservatives that allow yeasts to reproduce quickly.

## *Best Beverage Options*

Aside from practicing healthy eating habits, juicing (as well as making smoothies) also helps in building a strong immune system. The process of juicing allows your body to absorb vitamins and anti-oxidants in the purest form.

The ideal juice or smoothie is composed of 90% green vegetables and 10% fruits. Remember to keep your fruit intake low since it contains sugar.

These juicing recipes (they're mainly lists of fruits and vegetables, so simply mix the ingredients together in a blender) should help you get rid of your infection:

*Green Juice (aids in strengthening the immune system)*
- 2 cups spinach leaves
- 1 celery stalk
- ¼ cup lemon juice
- 1 clove garlic
- 1/2 cup water

*Mixed Veggie*
- 1 medium tomato
- 2 carrots
- 1 cup spinach leaves
- ½ cup parsley
- (Optional) add ½ cup water or several ice cubes

*Anti-Yeast Infection juice*
- 3 stalks celery
- 1 cucumber
- ¼ avocado
- 2 garlic cloves
- 1 small white onion
- You may add ½ cup water or ice cubes

*Avocado Green Smoothie*
- 1 medium avocado
- ½ green apple
- ¼ cup lemon juice
- 3 mint sprigs
- ¼ cup parsley leaves
- 1 cup water
- (Optional) add ½ cup plain yogurt

The recipes presented in here are simple to make. You will need a juicer or a blender to make these drinks. You have to incorporate as much green vegetables as possible in your drinks. Here's an extra tip – lemon juice is a good addition to any juice or smoothie recipe.

# A FINAL WORD

The best way to prevent the recurrence of yeast infection is to make some dietary changes (as suggested in the previous chapter) such as, avoidance of sugar, sugary foods and yeast-containing foods. You can also following a yeast free diet.

Keeping the genital area clean and dry, avoiding tight-fitting clothes and undergarments and drinking plenty of water throughout the day can prove helpful in this regard. However, be sure to inform your physician if the infection persists even after using the home remedies, and taking all possible preventive measures.

I want to take this time out to thank you for purchasing this book! The next step is to take action on the advice you've just read about.

## *Please Leave a Review*

Finally, if you enjoyed this book, please take the time to share your thoughts and post a review on Amazon. It'd be greatly appreciated!

That review and feedback will help me improve the content in my books – and make each and every one more relevant and helpful to you.

Thank you again and good luck!

Angie S